SIMPLIFY YOUR LIFE

TIPS FOR DEVELOPING A PURPOSE DRIVEN LIFE
AND UNLOCKING YOUR POTENTIAL

SARAH O'FLAHERTY

CONNECT THE DOTS

Get Sarah O'Flaherty's Online Values Lesson
FOR FREE

Join my VIP Club and get a free online values lesson, the simplify your life workbook, and the 12 steps to self-care poster, for free.

Details can be found at the end of this book.

PREFACE

Frustrated with the old processes of goal setting and outmoded self-help techniques, I've developed a new, simplified approach to personal development. This new methodology is not about striving, it's not about constant busyness, and it's not about the typical win-at-all-costs attitude.

This new system has been built from the integration of hundreds of books, a multitude of personal development training formats, many years of meditation and spiritual development, and a career based on motivating people and developing inspiring workplaces. At it's most basic, it has been built on a foundation of authenticity, simplicity, and genuine connection.

"I believe that each of us has our own path to follow. If we are walking this path, things flow, and we feel energized and happy."

~ Sarah O'Flaherty

Unfortunately, sometimes things happen in our lives that push us off track. It may be that we spend time working in a toxic environment, and instead of taking the hint that life is giving us, and changing jobs or careers, we stay in the negative environment, persist with it, hoping that things will get better. While persistence is a good quality, putting up with too much toxicity or wandering off our life path is not good at all. When we walk away from our 'yellow brick road' it can cause us to get sick, to take on some of the toxicity that surrounds us, and to put up barriers or unconscious blocks that aren't helpful for our future development.

Or maybe, you've spent years focusing on others; your children, your spouse, your friends, or your work colleagues. Again, this shows generosity of spirit, but if you've been so focused on others that you haven't been paying attention to yourself you may feel lost, like you're missing something, or maybe you just feel demotivated and lacking energy. You'll know when you're not acting in a way that's in alignment with your values. Taking some time out for you, and getting back on track will do wonders for your health and well-being, and will ensure you're more available for others in the longer term.

Here's a list of questions to assist you in deciding if this process is right for you:

Are you comfortable saying no?
Do you feel financially secure?
Do you feel that you know your life's purpose?
Are you living your values in all areas of your life?
Do you set healthy boundaries with others, especially those who are stressful to be around?
Do you consider yourself an optimist or a pessimist?
Are you in a positive relationship with a partner who allows you to be your true self?

Do you feel well supported by a loving community, good friends,
or a caring family?
Do you practice gratitude?
Do you do things to help others?
Are you able to deal with your negative emotions? And that
doesn't mean suppressing them.
Do you utilise relaxation and well-being techniques, such as
meditation, laughter, or mindfulness?
Do you express yourself creatively in ways you love?

This program is intended as a starting point to *reignite your passion for life.* You may take each section, and slowly work through it, moving on to the next one only once you feel comfortable with your progress at each stage. Or you can work through all the sections at once, and then go back and concentrate on areas you believe need more focus. You can also jump around a little, finding the chapters that most appeal and working on those to start with. Do whatever feels right for you. If you require additional assistance or would like to be coached through the process you can contact me at: sarah@sarahoflaherty.com.

To move through this process most effectively you need some undisturbed alone time. *This is time for YOU that should be free of distractions.* Why not go away for a weekend by yourself? Or, if you can't do that, then at least lock yourself in a room for a few hours at a time and ask your friends and family not to disturb you.

And try to keep the process light and fun – enjoy it! Life is an adventure and working through this process is only one part of the journey. I hope that by starting this adventure you'll discover new things about yourself. As you kick your creative brain into action, you may develop a new hobby or even become conscious of a passion that has been lying dormant within you.

By the end of this book, I hope you'll feel empowered and energised. There is a special kind of vibrancy that only comes from finding your own unique way in the world. Believe me, it really is worth taking the time to find your own special path.

PART I

LET'S TALK ABOUT YOU

1

IT'S ALL ABOUT YOU

You are the most important person in the room right now. Don't believe it? Really, you are! A few of you might be thinking, "Cool, I hope so." Yet, some of you will be thinking, "No way, not me!" It's very easy to fall into the trap of believing, "I'm not good enough, I'm not special, I don't know what my purpose is..." I know, I've been there myself. Even after a very successful career, and having lived a rather blessed life that has included living and working all around the world, I've often felt that I am somehow less than what I should be or could have been.

It took many years to change my own less than positive attitude, including a lot of meditation and mindfulness work, and reading a book that I highly recommend, called Love Yourself Like Your Life Depends on It by Kamal Ravikant. His inspiring story shows that in order to heal it is sometimes worthwhile to go to extremes. His recommendation to ask yourself, "If I loved myself truly and deeply, what would I do?" in any given situation, has been transformative for me.

Ultimately, you'll never be in any position to help others or even connect healthily with others if you are not comfortable with yourself. So, the first area of focus must be you.

2

BODY

"Treat your body like a temple, not a woodshed. The mind and the body work together. Your body needs to be a good support system for the mind and the spirit. If you take good care of it, your body can take you wherever you want to go, with the power and strength and energy and vitality you will need to get there."

~ Jim Rohn

I'm sure you know from your own experience that when your body is not functioning optimally it can impact your emotions and your thoughts. If you're not feeling well, it's very easy to feel grumpy and miserable. Of course, the other extreme is also true. When your body is in tip-top health, your emotions and thoughts seem to come along for the ride, and life is wonderful.

Your body is the foundation from which you operate, and treating your body like a temple means taking a holistic approach to your health. There is plenty of information around nowadays telling us to eat organic, cut out sugar, do this, don't do that. Sometimes it can be a little overwhelming, especially when you're already overloaded and overwhelmed with life. Where do you start?

To keep this fairly simple I've started with a quick health check and some suggestions on actions to take based on your result. Depending on your current level of health, your journey to optimal health may be a quick one, or it may require more time. If your health does need some work, then don't panic, and don't worry about how long it will take. Once your body starts healing it's amazing how quickly it seems to regenerate on its own. It seems to become an exponential process.

Below are some basic tips to get you going:

1. **Take in positive fuel.** Ideally, eat organic, locally grown, good food. Eliminate, or at least reduce, processed foods. If you question why you need to go organic rather than stick with conventionally farmed produce, the answer is simple. Organic foods have been proven to have more antioxidants than conventional foods, have a higher nutritional value, and significantly lower levels of pesticides (Andrews et al., 2008).
2. **Listen to your body.** Is that headache telling you to drink more coffee to perk you up, or is it saying slow down, drink some water, and take a rest. Take the time to listen to your body, don't just react with medications or quick fixes. Eat mindfully; notice what food makes you feel more energised, and what makes you feel agitated, sluggish, or grumpy.
3. **Get plenty of sleep.** It has been proven over and over

again that sleep is essential to ensure that the body and mind stay in top condition. Please don't buy into the hype that to be a high achiever you need to be doing, doing, doing, and sleeping only four hours a night. This is a media created fallacy. I don't know about you, but I used to read women's magazines and buy into the story of the successful businesswoman with a family who would get up at 5am to go to the gym, get her kids to school, work all day, and then have time to look glamorous and go out for a lovely boozy dinner with her friends until around midnight. These people are not real, please don't buy into the propaganda. To quote Matt Walker, an Associate Professor of Psychology at UC Berkeley and Principal Investigator at the Sleep and Neuro-Imaging Laboratory, "simply put, the single most important thing you can do each-and-every day to reset your brain and body health is to sleep. Once you start to get anything less than about seven hours of sleep, we can start to measure biological and behavioural changes quite clearly." Sleep is essential – again, you know what amount is best for you - but between seven to nine hours sleep a night is optimal.

4. **Stretch, strengthen, challenge.** We are all different, and our bodies require different levels and types of exercise, depending on our own unique makeup. Develop your own balance of stretching (e.g. yoga, tai chi), strengthening (e.g. weight training), and challenge (e.g. aerobic activity). These days there are unlimited exercise options – why not try to keep it fun? Another way to consider this option is to make sure that you have plenty of movement included in your daily schedule. Movement is particularly important if you're stuck in a desk job and find yourself at a computer all day. Walking meetings are increasing in popularity. When scheduling

your next meeting, particularly if it's with only one other person, why not make it a walking meeting? It's likely to be more fun, you'll get in a bit of movement, and you may even find that your brain clicks into a more creative mode and you come up with helpful solutions to problems quicker. Whatever your day looks like, get out there and go for a walk, take some time now, and move that body of yours.

5. **Reduce stress.** This modern day 'nasty' has become so prevalent in our society that millions of articles have been written on how to reduce the effects of stress. We generally use the word 'stress' when we feel that everything seems to have become too much. We feel overloaded and we wonder whether we can cope with the pressure we're feeling. When we feel stressed the following things happen to our body: blood pressure rises, breathing becomes more rapid, the digestive system slows down, heart-rate rises, immune system functioning goes down, muscles become tense, and we do not sleep well. In total, it's not good. There are many ways to deal with stress; talking to friends and family, taking time out for yourself, relaxation techniques – meditation, yoga, breathing, and seeking help from a professional. Don't let stress overtake you, it can and must be stopped before it does too much damage.

6. **Don't smoke, and go easy on the booze.** In many countries smoking is the single most preventable cause of illness and is a risk factor for lung cancer, emphysema, heart disease, and numerous other cancers. If you are a smoker, why not look at how you can quit? Go and see your doctor, they'll be able to fill you in on the best methods to use. Many people use alcohol to 'escape' from the stressors of their day, and yet, they forget that alcohol is a depressant. It slows the function of the

central nervous system and blocks messages trying to get to the brain. This point is simple really, don't smoke cigarettes and drink in moderation.

7. **Schedule regular 'me-time'** to de-stress and regroup. What you schedule for this time could be as simple as retreating to the tub for a long soak or playing a game of tennis with a friend. Or, it could be as indulgent as a weekend away at a spa. Do whatever works for you, and make sure you schedule it regularly. I recently did an Ayurvedic detox in Bali that was amazing. This type of detox is very gentle and is developed for your individual body type. I highly recommend this form of detoxing if you can find a good practitioner. Ideally, try to schedule in a detox program or a fast at least once a year. It can be done on retreat, or, if you have financial restrictions, then at home with friends can be another option. Although, do be aware that detoxing tends to bring out any emotional baggage you may have stored up. So, if you decide to do it with friends, ensure you have enough space to hide away for a while when you feel any strong emotions emerging.

8. **Slow down.** My final point is to try to slow down. Nearly all of us are operating at a very fast pace these days, and our breakneck speed adds to our stress and ensures that we miss what's happening day to day. I think you'll be surprised by the paradox that, as you slow down, time seems to expand. While you might think you'd get less done as you slow down, you often get more done, and each action becomes richer and more enjoyable. Try it for a day or two. Aim to do as little as possible, mindfully, and notice what you have completed by the end of the trial period.

One final comment to keep in mind as we continue this journey - as a life adventurer your body is the vessel that allows you to travel the oceans of this world. If you don't keep it watertight you may find yourself sinking rather than surfing the waves of life. Please, please, please take good care of your amazing beautiful body.

Workbook Exercise: Body Health

For the workbook exercises, you can write in this book if you have a hardcopy version, or you can buy a notebook to record your results, or, if you sign up to my VIP Club, you'll be sent the Simplify Your Life Workbook. Downloading the workbook or having a separate notebook are my recommendations, you'll have all your information in one spot, you can easily review your progress as you go, and you'll have extra paper for the insights and personal learnings that will emerge throughout the process.

Take a few minutes to rate how well you're looking after your body, and then, based on your score, follow the recommended action. Rate each of these elements on a scale of 1 to 10. 1 = "I'm a slacker" 10 = "I'm blitzing it"

- I eat mostly organic, locally grown food.
- I always listen to my body.
- I get plenty of sleep.
- I exercise regularly, in a way that suits my body type.
- I have good ways to handle stress.
- I don't drink alcohol or smoke.
- I schedule regular 'me-time'.
- I operate in the 'go slow' zone.

Total up your score, and then see where you sit below:

60-80: You're living the dream. You're very healthy and don't need to take any further action in this area of your life. You have a great foundation for moving forward.

40-60: You are fairly healthy. However, there are a few minor changes you could make to become invincible. See if there is any area that stands out as having a particularly low score and start making some changes there.

20-40: You need to work on this area of your life. Ideally, take the time to see a holistic health professional and get a full body check-up. You may need to make a lot of changes, and this can seem overwhelming at first. However, just choose one area at a time to work on before moving on to the next.

0-20: I hate to say this, but you're in trouble. Your health is not good. You need to take urgent action to get your body back to optimal health. See a health professional immediately.

3

MIND

You are not your mind, and you are most definitely not your thoughts. However, your mind is a part of you, a tool for you to utilise as you need. It's important that you look after it, ensure that you are in charge of it, and that it's not in charge of you.

You may feel as if you've walked into a science fiction novel here. How can my mind be in control of me? Isn't my mind just part of me? Am I being controlled by some kind of alien mind force? What the...? I know, I know, it all seems a little crazy. However, take a moment to think about it, your mind generates thousands and thousands of thoughts every day. In fact, on average, we each have around 70,000 thoughts a day. That's a lot of thoughts. How many of those thoughts are you aware of? Not 70,000, that's for sure. So, keeping that statistic in mind, I'm sure you can imagine how easy it can be for your mind to go into autopilot and for you to have little or no awareness of what you're thinking and doing.

Don't worry, I'm not implying that you can or should be aware of all your thoughts. However, if you aren't aware of any of them, or if you aren't aware of whether they're trending positive or negative, your mind may be more in control than you are. And that's not a good situation to be in. It's important to have a healthy mind, and an awareness of our thoughts and how they effect us. Below are a couple of tips that will help to ensure your mind stays healthy and assist you with keeping your thoughts in check.

1. **Keep the brain active.** It can be simple and enjoyable to challenge your mind, and in the process you are taking preventative action to ward off diseases such as Alzheimer's and Dementia. These challenges may take the shape of new physical skills - dancing or tennis, or mental exercises such as crossword puzzles, learning a new language, reading a challenging new book, or understanding a new computer system. By exercising your brain you are keeping it healthy and less susceptible to deterioration.

2. **Meditate.** It's good for you! And there's plenty of evidence to prove it. Many successful people, entrepreneurs, sportspeople, celebrities, are now regular meditators. It's a tool that more and more people are aware of and utilising to improve their lives. Here are just some of the benefits of meditation:

• Healing – decreased blood pressure and hypertension, lower cholesterol levels, improved immunity, reduced anxiety, and much more.

• Reducing stress and burnout – regular meditation

reduces accumulated stress and develops a state of
restful alertness.
- Enhancing concentration, memory and the ability to
learn – meditation is a powerful tool for awakening new
neural connections and even transforming regions of
the brain.

I am a big proponent of the practice of meditation and there are
plenty of resources, articles, and much more on my website if you
are interested in further information.

4

EMOTIONS

"If I feel depressed I will sing. If I feel sad I will laugh. If I feel ill I will double my labor. If I feel fear I will plunge ahead. If I feel inferior I will wear new garments. If I feel uncertain I will raise my voice. If I feel poverty I will think of wealth to come. If I feel incompetent I will think of past success. If I feel insignificant I will remember my goals. Today I will be the master of my emotions."

~ Og Mandino

In the same way that you are not your mind or your thoughts, you are also not your emotions. The key to managing our emotions is becoming aware of them, noticing them as soon as they arise. A friend of mine who used to be a Buddhist monk in Thailand used this analogy to explain emotions - your emotions are like a fire in a forest, if you get too close to the fire you will get burnt, but if you don't keep an eye on the fire, it could very quickly burn out of control.

What is extremely helpful in assisting with the management of emotions is the practice of mindfulness. When an emotion arises, put your attention on it, don't buy into the story surrounding the emotion, and definitely don't add fuel to the fire. Bringing your awareness to your emotions before they take over your body can be challenging, however, its worth working on. Once you're aware of your emotions you'll notice that they do not grow, they do not become more intense, you can, at the very least, get them into a holding pattern. In this way you can be certain that you won't encourage the fire to turn into a raging bonfire that needs the fire brigade to come and put it out.

When noticing the emotion, the following questions may help. How does it make your body feel? Hot, cold, agitated? Where is the feeling located in your body? Does it make you feel good or bad? Spend some time understanding your emotions. Notice what negative emotions arise regularly, and also notice what positive emotions you feel most often. We all tend to act quite habitually, so it's not surprising that the same emotional patterns tend to come up over and over again. As you understand your emotions better you will be better able to keep them under control.

Don't judge or blame yourself for your emotions. We are all human, and emotions are part of our make-up. They usually come up for a reason, and they need to be processed and released. They only become damaging when we let them take over, and we act out certain behaviours that may cause damage to others or ourselves.

" *Negative emotions like loneliness, envy, and guilt have an important role to play in a happy life; they're big, flashing signs that say something needs to change.*"

~ *Gretchen Rubin*

I'd like to take a moment to talk about the negative emotions, in particular, envy. Now, I know you might be wondering, why on earth do I want to talk about envy? It's a horrible negative emotion, isn't it, one we're not supposed to have? And yet, a presentation I saw by the renowned philosopher Alain de Botton, got me thinking about envy and how it can be really useful. I hope that this example will help you to see how all our emotions can be useful whether they are negative or positive.

In Alain's talk, about the media and it's influence on our lives, he outlined how we are taught in our Judeo-Christian society that envy is very bad, and yet we all feel envy all the time. Alain suggests that we use our envy to help us. He mentions keeping an envy diary where you write down every time you feel envious, noting who made you envious and why. Because "envy is like a scattered jigsaw of your future self, inside every envious attack is a clue as to who you should be, but have not yet become. Often the clues are a bit weird, and a bit misleading, so you have to filter through the fog, you have to analyse your envy, but it is a set of clues. So don't sit on your envy and pretend it doesn't exist. Look at it and analyse it" (de Botton, 2014).

By following Alain's advice, you may find that what you're actually envious of is not the wealth or success of the other person, but their courage, for example. So you discover that what you want to develop in yourself is increased levels of courage. After listening to this talk I started my own envy diary and it's been very insightful and rather useful. First, you identify whom you envy in the world, and then, what it is about them that you envy – look deeply, go past the first impressions. You start to see very clearly what's important to you and you discover the character

traits of others that you'd like to become part of your make-up.
Try it out for yourself, it's fun.

SELF-AWARENESS

"Your visions will become clear only when you can look into your own heart. Who looks outside, dreams; who looks inside, awakes."

~ *C.G. Jung*

Self-awareness is important. When we have a better understanding of ourselves, we are able to truly experience what unique individuals we are. We become empowered to make changes and to build on our areas of strength, as well as identify areas where we would like to make improvements. Self-awareness is being conscious of what you're good at, while acknowledging what you still have to learn.

Let's start with values. What are your values? They are those things that you believe are important to the way you operate in the world. They help you determine your priorities. You can consider them the signposts that provide direction in your life. There is a very good reason why identifying your values is the first step in ensuring you know yourself, because your values impact everything; who you have relationships with, where you work, and even where you're investing your money for your retirement. If you get clear on your values and ensure your life is aligned with them, you'll find that your energy levels lift and your life moves into a synergistic flow. When the things that you do, and the way you behave, match your values, life is usually good – you're satisfied and content. But when your actions don't align with your values, that's when things feel and can go very wrong. Making a conscious effort to identify your values is very important.

Workbook Exercise: Values List

In the Appendix you'll find a list of values. Review all the values listed, select your top 10, and note them down in your workbook. The next step is to narrow this list down to five, and again list these in your workbook.

Top Ten Values:

1. _____
2. _____
3. _____
4. _____
5. _____
6. _____
7. _____
8. _____
9. _____

10._____

Top Five Values:

1. _____
2. _____
3. _____
4. _____
5. _____

Congratulations! You've discovered your top five values.

Once you know your values, it's also helpful to identify your strengths. Strengths are tasks or actions you do well. How well do you know your strengths? Strengths are often those things that come most naturally to us. Research shows that using our strengths makes us happier, especially if we can find new ways to implement them.

Workbook Exercise: Strengths

The easiest way to determine your strengths is to do an online survey. There are many of these now readily available for free. One I can recommend is the University of Pennsylvania VIA Survey of Character Strengths. You'll first need to register, it's free and they don't spam you, and then go to the questionnaires section and do the VIA Survey of Character Strengths.

The results will show you which of the 24 character strengths are your 'signature strengths'. Make sure you answer each question as you are now, not how you think you should be or would like to be. Even if you think you know your top strengths I highly recommend you give this survey a try and see what results show up for you. You may be surprised to find you have a strength that you hadn't been consciously aware of before. Once you've completed the survey, and received the results, list down your top five strengths.

Top Five Strengths:

1. _____
2. _____
3. _____
4. _____
5. _____

When you have your top five strengths listed, take some time to review them. Look at each one and ask yourself – do I feel naturally drawn to this strength? Does it excite and energise me? Do I feel surprised by it? Is it real for me? How much do I use this strength (at home, at work)? Do others see this strength in me? If you're struggling to answer these questions on your own, you can ask your friends and family for their input.

If you're not comfortable with one of the top five strengths in your list then review numbers six, seven, and eight. Relook at the questions listed above and get to a list of five that you really feel you can own. Next ask yourself, "how are you using these strengths in your life? Where are you using them? In what other areas in your life could you use them more?" Over the next week try to use one of your strengths in a new way, or in a new area of your life. Each week take a little bit of time to work on a different strength. As I mentioned earlier, implementing your strengths has been proven to increase happiness, so I'd suggest it's time to get working your strength muscles.

Next up are passions, do you know your passions? Identifying your passions may be easy for you. What do you love doing? What do you spend your time doing when you are totally free to choose what you want to do? What gives you energy? Or, maybe you have no idea what your passions are, no problem, this is not unusual. Most people don't know what their passions are. Many of us had passions when we were younger that we've forgotten, or we may have been told they were silly, or that they wouldn't ensure a socially acceptable career, so we let them go, or were encouraged to move on to other things.

Workbook Exercise: Passions

To live a passionate life, it's important to identify what your passions are and start doing them. Then, whether you use your passions for work or play, you'll find that your life is fuller and more energised. If you already know your passions then list them down. If you're not sure, then ask yourself the following questions to see what comes up for you:

What are my goals?
If I could do one thing for the rest of my life, what would it be?

What would I love to try?
What have I never done before that I'd love to do?
What would I do, even if I didn't get paid to do it?
What makes me feel like nothing else exists?
What activity makes me feel completely in my element?
When do I feel 'in the zone' or when does time disappear?

Hopefully, these questions helped get your creative juices flowing. But if you're still stuck then here are some more:

What is the one thing I've always dreamed about doing, but
haven't done yet?
What did I want to do when I was a child?
What subjects did I love at school?
Do I have an impractical dream that I once abandoned?
Is there something I've been afraid to try because it takes me out
of my comfort zone?
Is there something I've always wanted to do but haven't done
because of financial fears?
Is there something I've always wanted to do but haven't tried
because I've been afraid I'd fail or just not be very good at it?
Is there something that someone I know does that thrills me?

My Passions

1. _____
2. _____
3. _____

4. _____

5. _____

I hope you now have enough material to complete a list of passions.

What do you feel is missing in your life right now? What is important to you that you're not getting? These missing factors could be emotional, for example, respect. Or, it may be something you'd like to be doing that you just can't seem to find the time for, for example, meditation. Identifying what is missing in your life helps you to see if there are any gaps that need some attention.

Workbook Exercise: Missing

Identify what you feel is missing in your life. Do you want more love? Do you want more time to yourself? Review the following aspects of your life and see if there is anything missing for you:

Relationships, career and business, finance, health and well-being, personal development, free/fun time, contribution/spirituality

Missing

I. _____

2. _____

3. _____

4. _____

5. _____

~

Yes, self-awareness is a big section, and I still have more questions. Are you an introvert or an extrovert? You may think this a
strange question, but it's important to know which modality you
operate within to be sure you are doing what's best for you. I
recently read a book that fundamentally changed my view of the
world and myself. To be honest, I wish it had been available 20
years ago when I was at university and deciding on a career path.
Whether you think you're an introvert or an extrovert this book is
well worth a read. The book is called Quiet: The Power of Introverts in a World That Can't Stop Talking by Susan Cain.

The excerpt below is from Susan Cain's Website:

*Why does it matter where you fall on the introvert-extrovert spectrum?
Because introversion and extroversion are at the heart of human
nature. And when you make life choices that are congruent with your
temperament, you unleash vast stores of energy.*

*Conversely, when you spend too much time battling your own nature,
the opposite happens—you deplete yourself. Too many people live lives
that don't suit them—introverts with frenetic social schedules, extroverts with jobs that require them to sit in front of their computers for
hours at a stretch. We all have to do things that don't come naturally—
some of the time. But it shouldn't be all the time. It shouldn't even be
most of the time.*

Remember, though, that no one is all introvert or all extrovert. Intro-

verts attend wild parties, and extroverts curl up with their favourite books. As the psychologist Carl Jung put it, "There is no such thing as a pure extrovert or a pure introvert. Such a man would be in the lunatic asylum."

It's a bit of fun to do her 10-question test to see where you fall on the introvert-extrovert scale.

SELF-ACCEPTANCE

"When you take charge of your life, there is no longer a need to ask permission of other people or society at large. When you ask permission, you give someone veto power over your life."

~ Geoffrey F. Abert

It's important to be comfortable with who you are, remember no-one's perfect. Unfortunately, we frequently compare ourselves to others, dwelling on our flaws - what we're *not* rather than what we've *got*. And it's this type of thinking that makes it so much harder to be happy. Learning to accept ourselves, warts and all, and being kinder to ourselves when things go wrong, increases our enjoyment of life, our resilience, and our well being. It also helps us to accept others as they are.

Well-rounded people are not ashamed or guilty about their human nature, with its shortcomings, imperfections, frailties, and weaknesses. Nor are they critical of these aspects of other people.

They respect and esteem themselves and others. And this helps them to be open, honest, and genuine, without pose or façade.

Workbook Exercise: Self-Acceptance

A very helpful self-acceptance exercise is to list all your good qualities and I have absolutely no doubt that you have plenty of amazing traits. Let's get them all down on paper. If you struggle with this exercise, and some of us are not very good at seeing the best in ourselves, then ask friends and family what they consider your positive qualities to be.

My Positive Qualities:

1. _____
2. _____
3. _____
4. _____
5. _____
6. _____
7. _____
8. _____
9. _____
10. _____

Take the time to review your list. Really notice and appreciate all your good qualities. We all find it very easy to be self-critical, and strangely, it's not often that we're self-complimentary. So, enjoy this focus on the positive for a change. One way to get this exercise to sink in is, if you feel up for it, to look at yourself in the mirror and say, "I am...", and list off all your good qualities. Do it slowly and appreciate each compliment as it comes. A word of warning, I've had a few people tell me that this exercise has bought them to tears, good tears, but tears all the same. It's a powerful exercise and may be worth doing daily if you are struggling with accepting yourself as you are.

Another benefit of this exercise is that when negative thoughts about yourself come up, as soon as they come up, remember the good qualities you have listed here, and do the exercise above if you need to. Keep focusing on the positive, and you'll find the more negative thoughts and perceptions will fade. Thinking bad things about yourself doesn't do anyone any good – least of all you. I am very aware that too many of us focus on the negative and spend too much time beating ourselves up about being imperfect human beings, when really, that's exactly what we are, and it's what we're meant to be, wonderful interesting imperfect creatures.

To sum up the 'Let's talk about you' section, we've talked about the importance of looking after your body, your mind, and managing your emotions. By becoming more self-aware, you should now be able to identify your values, your strengths, your passions, what's missing in your life, and whether you're more of an introvert or extrovert. You'll also be more aware of the importance of self-acceptance, understanding what your positive qualities are and the importance of integrating those qualities into your being. This is a great start, and I hope it's lifted your energy levels at least a little.

PART II

LET'S TALK ABOUT YOU AND ME

7

THE IMPORTANCE OF RELATIONSHIPS

Knowing yourself is critical, and understanding how you interact with others is the next most important thing to consider. It is only possible to truly know ourselves when we are in relationship with others. You can see how true this statement is if we just think about our emotions for a moment. It is very rare that we get angry or upset when we are alone. However, when we are with others our buttons get pushed and we can get angry, upset, and confused. It's at these times when we need to work hard on what has triggered us, how we relate to the triggering person, and how to keep our relationships healthy and strong. This section takes a close look at the people you are spending time with, how you're interacting with others, and offers some relationship strategies that you may find helpful.

TRIBE

"I know there is strength in the differences between us. I know there is comfort, where we overlap."

~ Ani DiFranco

A tribe is a group of people with a common character, occupation, or interest. We're all part of many tribes; our families, groups of friends, work colleagues, to name just a few. Those whom we associate with, in part, define us, and this can be a good or a bad thing depending on whether our groups, or tribes, match our values and needs, and whether they have a positive or negative influence on us.

Our tribes provide us with a sense of belonging and community, and they can be extremely helpful in supporting our needs and values. For example, if you're trying to change your eating habits, say to cut out sugar, then it helps to be part of a community that provides you with tips and ideas on how to achieve that change. It can also be helpful if you have a friend who decides to make the change at the same time as you. You can support each other with your daily and weekly wins, discuss moments of weakness, and develop strategies to ensure they don't happen again.

One of the benefits of the internet is the proliferation of online communities. These communities connect you to people with similar interests where you can share ideas, ask questions, and gain support. No matter who you are, or where you're located in the world, you can join an online community that suits you. Let's use the example mentioned above, cutting out sugar. There are many online communities you can join to help you in this endeavour. Two interesting ones that are worth checking out are: Sarah Wilson's – I Quit Sugar, and Dr. Junger's – Clean. While online communities are great, it will always be important to have real live face-to-face connections as well. In this example, you may want to see your local doctor for support, or you may connect with a good friend who you know is also interested in improving their health and well-being. The social support structure you establish, and how strong it is, could be the 'make or break' of your new mission.

Unfortunately, sometimes we belong to tribes that have a negative influence in our lives. It may be that we are part of a community that doesn't suit our values. For example, you join a book club because you're interested in books and reading, and yet, after a couple of meetings it becomes clear to you that the focus of the meeting is drinking wine and gossiping, two things you don't really enjoy. However, you like the people and it's kind of fun, so you keep going, but when you look back after a few months of meetings you realise that you're now drinking more when you were trying to drink less, and it's set you off smoking again – damn it! So you can see how easy it is to fall in with the wrong tribe, and how quickly they can have a negative influence on your behaviour.

At this point, you need to consider whether it's really working for you to be part of this particular tribe. Do you want to continue for the social benefits, and stop drinking and smoking when you attend? Or do you want to find a new group that really is passionate about books and good conversation? Don't get me wrong. I'm not against wine and having fun. But sometimes the reason we get into things eventually doesn't correlate with what's actually happening in the group. It's important to regularly review the tribes we're part of and consciously decide whether they really suit us or not.

Workbook Exercise: Your Tribe

List the tribes you're part of, you can use the categories listed below or make up your own. Take some time to think through all the areas of your life where you're connected to others. Are you part of a movie club or book club? Are you on a social committee at work? List down whatever tribes you can think of.

Once you've listed all the tribes you're part of, then decide whether they're having a positive or negative influence on your life. For any tribes that are negative, you need to consider whether you should leave the group, or if there is an alternative solution. Using the book club example, can you have a discussion with the group and see if they'll refocus on books, or do you feel it is a lost cause and you'd rather find another book club to join. It's up to you to decide.

- Family/Relationships
- Career/Business

- Financial
- Health & Well-being
- Personal Development
- Free/Fun Time
- Contribution/Spirituality

9

CONNECTION

"I define connection as the energy that exists between people when they feel seen, heard, and valued; when they can give and receive without judgment; and when they derive sustenance and strength from the relationship."

~ *Brene Brown*

These days it's easy to think we have friends all over the world, especially with Facebook and other social mediums keeping us connected. But how many real friends do you have? Not online friends, not acquaintances, but those people you see face-to-face regularly, or at least Skype with regularly if you're an incessant traveler like me. Who are those people whose birthdays you remember, those people you really care about and who really care about you? I mean, really, how many people can you call at 1am to get you out of a jam?

In ancient times, before Facebook and mobile phones – yes, I was around then - you used to have to be at home by the phone (an old-fashioned landline phone) to talk to your friends when you weren't with them. I'm talking about back in the '80s. At that time, according to a few articles I've read, we had an average of three friends each. These days things have changed quite dramatically, we now operate very differently, we can meet whomever we like, whenever we like. We seem to have millions of friends – all our Facebook friends, our professional connections on LinkedIn, the friends we communicate with by text, and many more. However, do these extensive networks really mean that we have more friends? Or do we only appear to be more connected?

Conveniently, some very smart people have done studies to see how many friends we can realistically manage. One of those smart people is Professor Robin Dunbar who, in the early 1990's, proposed Dunbar's number. This number is the suggested cognitive limit of the number of people with whom we can maintain stable social relationships. These are relationships in which an individual knows who each person is, and how each person relates to every other person in the group. Through a number of experiments he proposed that humans could only comfortably maintain 150 stable relationships. Now that's a big number. You may be thinking, really, we've gone from three to 150? Initially, that does seem like a lot of people, but Dunbar then breaks the 150 people down into distinct groups.

In the study, Dunbar states that we are only able to maintain an inner circle of about five close friends – these are your best friends, the ones you can call anytime to get you out of a 'fix.' Next on the hierarchy are 10 friends - those you'd invite to your housewarming party or a very large dinner party. Then there are the next 35, we'll call this group your extended circle of friends, those people from sports groups, work, etc. The final 100 are really just acquaintances, perhaps the staff at your local supermarket, or your local policeman, people you know by name and would chat with on the street, but you wouldn't necessarily invite around to your house for dinner. And there are your 150.

So, in reality, we've gone from three to five good friends. It's not that big a leap is it? And, doesn't it make you wonder – who are all those people you're friends with on Facebook? How many of those people have you communicated with outside of Facebook? How many of them are really your friends? How many of those people could you call to get you out of a jam? In conclusion, and to support Dunbar's theory, I found this wonderful old Portuguese saying, and it's so true:

"You have five friends, and the rest is landscape."

Workbook Exercise: Connection

The purpose of this exercise is to bring your closest friends into conscious awareness. As with all the exercises in this book, the aim is to bring the simple aspects of your life into your awareness so you can consciously decide if they are right for you or not. I'd like to point out that you shouldn't consider these lists as set in stone, our friends may vary and change over our lifetime.

List down your top five friends, then list your next 10.

Top Five Friends

1. _____
2. _____
3. _____
4. _____
5. _____

Next Ten Friends

I. _____

2. _____

3. _____

4. _____

5. _____

6. _____

7. _____

8. _____

9. _____

10. _____

How are you prioritising your time and energy in relation to your friends? Do you know who your close friends are? Do you spend most of your time and energy on or with them? Are you spending some time with your outer circle of friends and only limited time with your acquaintances?

You may also want to do some connection expansion work every now and then. Are there any people you'd like to connect with more? Because our relationships change and vary over time, it's always healthy to develop some new relationships during your life adventure.

Relook at your list of friends now. Make sure you are happy with your list and then pour your energy into those relationships.

WISE FRIENDS

"An insincere and evil friend is more to be feared than a wild beast; a wild beast may wound your body, but an evil friend will wound your mind."

~ *Buddha*

Please excuse the rather dramatic quote, but I wanted to grab your attention and I must admit, it also provides some very good advice. Too often we just fall in with a group of friends not thinking much about the process or who those people are. We meet them somewhere, we do a few things together, and then we just start hanging out. How much time did we actually spend considering whether they fit with our values, whether they are a good or bad influence, whether they add to our energy levels or whether they seem to drain away our energy reserves?

I can speak from experience here. I seem to make friends very easily, which has made all my moving around rather straightforward. However, this has sometimes meant that I have found myself attached to some not particularly supportive people, and even infrequently to some rather 'bad eggs.' I know that the people I associate with influence me, and when I've been hanging with those 'bad eggs,' I'll admit that at times I haven't behaved my best. Perhaps you've had a similar experience? The opposite is also true. When I'm with people I find wise and inspiring I seem to function at a higher level, I become my best self. These days, I'm not so easily influenced, and I spend most of my time with those I consider wise friends.

Workbook Exercise: Wise Friends

When considering your list of close friends from the previous exercise, review the questions below for each person. You can answer each question with a tick or a cross, or with words, whatever suits you. Hopefully, you'll find that most of your friends are adding value to your life. Remember that no-one is perfect, but if you have any friends that seem to be having more of a negative than positive impact on your life, then you need to consider if they are really the kind of people you want to associate with.

1. Values: Do you have the same or similar values?
2. Balance: Do you tend to help each other out in a balanced way? Are you driving the relationship? Is your friend? Or is your relationship and communication balanced?
3. Advice: Does your friend give you good or wise advice most of the time?

Of course, this is not an exhaustive list of all the qualities of friends, but it will give you a good indication of whether your friends are a positive or negative influence in your life. Feel free to make up your own checklist – there may be some qualities that are not listed here that are very important to you. It's very important to always do what's right for you.

After working through this section, how do you feel about how you are in relationship? Are you part of a strong healthy tribe? They are your community and support networks. How well are you connected? Do you know who your close friends are? Make sure you're not spreading yourself too thinly and trying to be best friends with everyone in the world. And remember, we all have some friends that we do not see or connect with for years, and yet when we catch up with them it seems that no time has passed and we're back at the same wonderful place as the last time we met. Don't forget these friends. You might even want to make a separate list for them - your wonderful long-term friends who you may not see very often because they live overseas or are busy with family. And finally, are your friends wise friends? Be sure that you have friends that support you and meet you at a values level.

PART III

LET'S TALK ABOUT ALL THE GOOD THINGS AND THE BAD THINGS

11

HOW DO YOU RELATE TO THE WORLD?

First there's you, then there's you and others, and finally, there's taking a bigger perspective and including the whole world. To live a full life you need to go beyond yourself. This includes being aware of the environment you are operating in, using creativity to broaden your outlook, taking time to explore the world - to try new things, and finding your purpose - understanding how you can be of service in the world. This is the really fun bit! We've done the foundational work, and now we're building our castle. To live the life we dream of we need to get a little adventurous and take charge of our kingdom.

12

ENVIRONMENT

"Your outlook upon life, your estimate of yourself, your estimate of your value are largely coloured by your environment. Your whole career will be modified, shaped, moulded by your surroundings, by the character of the people with whom you come in contact every day."

~ Orison Swett Marden

Whether we like it or not, we're all affected by our environment. Since the beginning of time, human beings have needed to be sensitive to their surroundings in order to survive, we have an innate awareness of our environment and we seek out certain qualities in our habitat. The three main conditions we tend to focus on are:

1. Safety and security
2. Physical comfort – e.g. not too hot, and not too cold

3. Psychological comfort – e.g. environments that are familiar, but offer the right amount of stimulus.

Below are just a few examples of how your environment can impact you:

- Environments can facilitate or discourage interactions among people. For example, an inviting space with comfortable chairs encourages social interaction.
- Environments can influence people's behaviour and motivation to act. For example, it has been proven that a house that is in disrepair is more likely to be a target for vandalism than one that is well looked after.
- Environments can influence mood. For example, have you noticed how much better you feel in a room filled with natural light versus one lit with fluorescents.

Perhaps most importantly for health, environments can create or reduce stress, which in turn impacts our bodies in multiple ways. This impact occurs because our brain, our nervous system, our endocrine system, and our immune system, are constantly interacting. As neuroscientist Candice Pert puts it, "What you are thinking at any moment is changing your biochemistry." Thus, the stress of a noisy, confusing environment may result in you feeling worried, sad, or helpless, and experiencing changes to your body such as higher blood pressure, heart rate, and muscle tension.

Experts have identified five environmental attributes that can have a large impact on health outcomes.

1. **Increased connection to nature.** Many studies provide strong evidence that even three to five minutes of contact

with nature can significantly reduce stress and have a complex impact on emotions, reducing anger and fear, and increasing pleasant feelings. The Berman et al. (2008) study showed that adults received a mental boost after an hour-long walk in a woodland park – improving their performance on memory and attention tests by 20 per cent – compared to those who took an hour-long stroll in a noisy urban environment. Additionally, the Bowler et al. (2010) review that covered 25 relevant studies, found that exposure to a natural environment rather than a more synthetic setting showed a positive health benefit. Just one of these benefits was reduced negative emotions, such as anger and sadness. It's interesting, as I look out my window now all I can see are the tops of beautiful green trees, and there is nothing more refreshing and rejuvenating for me than that amazing view. And, as the trees sway and dance in the wind, I get the sense that the trees are with me on my journey, I never feel totally alone when connected to nature. Take a moment to think about how you feel when you are in nature, is it not grounding, restorative, and re-energising for you too?

2. **Options and choices.** Your ability to control your environment can significantly lessen stress. When you are in an environment where the lighting is too strong, and you can't change it, you'll feel stressed. Unfortunately, this is often the case in hospitals. However, when you are in an environment where you have control over adjustable elements such as music, lighting, and heat levels, you'll find yourself much happier and far less stressed.

3. **Close support.** There is extensive evidence that the social support of family and close friends has important health benefits. An example of this would be if you've just had a child, it will make a huge difference to you if

you have a supportive family nearby or if your family lives far away.

4. **Reduced environmental stressors such as noise, glare, and poor air quality.** Noise causes stress, as evidenced by increased heart rate and blood pressure, and reduced oxygen levels in the blood in both adults and babies. Glare and poor air quality are other environmental stressors. Consider whether any of these external environmental stressors are impacting you, because if it can be removed it will reduce stress.

5. **Pleasant diversions.** An aesthetically pleasing environment helps to reduce anxiety and stress. Such diversions may include: artwork of nature (not abstract art), fireplaces, videos of nature, and aquariums.

Workbook Exercise: Environment

Let's take a look at how well your environment suits you. For any environment you find yourself in, check how it ranks in the following areas:

1. Safety and security
2. Physical comfort
3. Psychological impact

Here are a few questions you can ask yourself:

Home:
Where do you live?
How is the energy?

Do you have enough space?
What is your neighbourhood like?
Is your home quiet or are you impacted by outside noise?

Work:
How is your work environment?
Is it healthy?
Is it safe?
Do people treat each other well?
Are you getting natural light?
Are you sitting all day or are you able to move around?

Consider what can and can't be changed. Can you make any of your environments more suited to what you need? Write down your thoughts and inspirations in your workbook.

13

CREATIVITY

"Everyone is born creative; everyone is given a box of crayons in kindergarten. Then when you hit puberty they take the crayons away and replace them with dry, uninspiring books on algebra, history, etc. Being suddenly hit years later with the 'creative bug' is just a wee voice telling you, 'I'd like my crayons back, please."

~ Hugh MacLeod

Creative output affects our ability to live a fulfilling life. Taking perhaps overly simplistic view of the brain as a way to conceptualise the difference between creativity and logic, the left side of the brain is often referred to as being more adept at tasks that involve logic, language, and analytical thinking. It is the part of the brain that deals with numbers and reasoning, it tends to be the side of the brain that we use most often in our daily life. Whereas, the right side of the brain is considered to be the creative and expressive part, it is the part that is associated with emotions, colour, images, music, intuition and even recognising faces. I've found, the more I tap into my creative, expressive, intuitive side, and let my logical, rational side take a break, the lighter and happier I feel.

Creativity is an aspect of self that many people ignore. It may seem that creativity is not what we need to get through our day, it may not be where the money is, and yet, there is a part in all of us that is creative, and that part needs to express itself. You may already know where your creative passion lies. Maybe you discovered it in the passions section of this book. Maybe you play the guitar, and just don't do it enough. Or, if you're not sure what your passion is yet, don't worry, it's great fun to try out a few things and see what suits you best. And a little side-note here, journaling is a very creative exercise with the added bonus of being very cathartic – writing in a journal has been proven to make you feel better. It's a great daily habit to pick up. As well as improving your writing skills, you'll find that getting everything down on paper helps to clear your head, and it can take a lot of the emotion out of difficult situations. If you're having a challenging day, or you have a challenging situation to deal with, don't forget to try a little journaling.

Before we move on to the workbook exercise I want to talk a little bit about play and the importance of taking the time to have some fun. For some reason play is generally viewed as only relevant to young children, and something you must give up as you grow older. Perhaps you feel that it's slightly dangerous to even consider playing as an adult, isn't work the respectable thing we should be filling our time with, not play? We have another misconception about play, that play is easy, which is not at all true. As adults we can engage in some very difficult and challenging activities when we play, for example, during sports, while playing music, and developing strategies in games like chess (Csikszentmihalyi, 1990). Another misconception we have, is that play is irrelevant or inconsequential, when in fact, it's actually very important and useful. It's a shame we've created all these falsities, as play has been found to be an important mediator for learning and socialisation throughout our lives (Csikszentmihalyi, 1990).

There are many benefits to play; it can help us to learn something new and useful, it can improve and enable our social needs, it can fulfil our need for competition, it can liberate the mind to allow for more creative and imaginative thinking, it can help us to achieve optimal life experiences, and it can increase our level of enjoyment, which has intrinsic worth of it's own (Rieber, 1996). So don't forget to play a little – just have fun! And you can lose the guilt because you know it's good for you!

Workbook Exercise: Creativity

Go to your workbook and get ready to get creative. If you already know what your creative outlet is then schedule it in to your diary at regular times each week. If you don't know what your creative passion is yet, then check out the list below and see if anything inspires you.

Photography
Drawing
Painting
Writing
Learning guitar, piano, saxophone, etc.
Cooking
Gardening
Making jewellery
Pottery
Singing

Dancing

Once you've found something, and it may not necessarily be on this list, find out where you can give it a try. Maybe a community college near you is offering lessons? Check out meet-up groups online, and see if there is a group you can join. If you look hard enough, you'll find some way to give it a go. And, please don't say that you don't have time. You have time, this is important and it will make a big difference to your life!

14

EXPLORATION

"Man cannot discover new oceans unless he has the courage to lose sight of the shore."

~ Andre Gide

Another important facet of being a human is that we have a never-ending urge to grow and evolve. You may have heard of Maslow's Hierarchy of Needs, this hierarchy reveals that our needs can be categorised into different levels, we must be fulfilled at each level before we can move up to the next one. The first level of needs are basic physiological needs – food, drink, sex, and sleep. These are the basics we require to survive. The second level includes the needs of safety and security, both physically and economically. The hierarchy works its way up to level five which equates to self-actualisation - our ability to reach our full personal potential. This level is the desire to accomplish every-thing that one can, to become the most that one can be. Our desires vary greatly, for one person their ultimate desire may be to become the perfect parent, for another it may be to become a famous painter. In order to get to this level, one must not only achieve all the previous levels, but one must master them. The level below self-actualisation is self-esteem. Self-esteem reflects a person's value of their worth, and can include positive or negative evaluations. Self-esteem is considered by some to be a combination of self-confidence and self-respect. A good way to work on our self-esteem is through exploration. Trying new things out, understanding what we are good at, what we are not so good at, what we love to do, and what is totally not for us.

Make your life richer by learning something new or trying new things. Try a new food; something exotic, let the new taste sensations take you on a journey to where that recipe came from. Try a new workout; give your body an energy boost by trying something totally different, you may notice muscles that you hadn't felt before, you may get into a flow that you hadn't experienced before, and you may find a new regime that works for you. There are plenty of benefits to exploring – it opens your mind, broadens your horizon, and often introduces you to new people.

I'm a natural explorer, it's just in my genes, and I explore in many ways - through learning, writing, experimenting - but, I have to admit that my main form of exploring is travel. I absolutely love to travel – to go to different places, to meet new people, to taste new foods. Traveling makes my soul sing. Why don't you find out what makes your soul sing?

Workbook Exercise: Exploration

How much exploration are you doing now? Are you learning/growing? What new things did you learn in the last year, in the last month? List them down.

If your list is looking a little light, then I suggest you be brave, step out of your comfort zone and try at least one new thing this month. It doesn't have to be massive or expensive – just trying a new dish with the right perspective can make a big difference to your life. Below are a few questions to help you with this exercise.

How do you step outside your comfort zone?
Are there things you'd like to learn or try?
Do you take different routes to work each day?
Have you met anyone new lately?
Would you like to learn a new language?

15

PURPOSE/MEANING

He who has a why to live for can bear almost any how."

~ *Friedrich Nietzsche*

Another purpose quote I love comes from Guru Singh, "The only way that you are going to succeed in your mission here on earth is to stop reacting to the majority and focus on your purpose." How do you find your purpose? That is the BIG question. It's a question that is important to find the answer to, because once you find your purpose you really are in heaven, you've found your reason for being in the world. Your purpose is often to do with how you can best serve others. Once you're living on purpose, you'll observe your energy levels pick up, you'll find life more fun, and you won't be able to wait for each new day to start.

However, once you've found your purpose, it isn't necessarily totally smooth sailing to start with. Finding your purpose and sticking with it is tough, and it's important to be aware of this up front so you can face the challenges as they come along. I remember reading about J. K. Rowling, the famous Harry Potter author, really struggling before she reached the great heights of fame and fortune. At one stage she was on the welfare benefit, and about as poor as it was possible to be in Britain without being homeless. She was frequently told early on in her writing career not to give up her day job as it was unlikely that she would make money from her children's books. Luckily, she felt compelled to write the Harry Potter books, and was determined to continue on with them no matter what challenges she faced along the way. And look at her now – she's a high-profile celebrity and one of the richest women in the UK.

Be aware that many of those successful artists, actors, business people, and community leaders who we now see at the top of their game once had to go through this challenging process too. They all had to take the time to figure out their purpose, and once they discovered it, they too had to go through many ups and downs and hardships to get to where they are now. So, when you face a tough patch, just remember those people at the top of their game faced similar challenges and proved that overcoming them was worth the effort.

Another thing that's worth remembering is that your calling chooses you. It's something that draws you, that drives you, and it pulls at you until you listen and start taking action. There's something very appealing about your calling choosing you. I like it because I believe it helps us to drop the 'I'm the one in control here' persona, and relax into the process of finding our purpose.

Unfortunately, many of us have been trained out of the idea that we can live a life full of passion and purpose. We might have a creative purpose, but were told early in life that creativity will never earn us enough money to survive. Or, we're just stuck in the rat-race cycle of work, spend, work, spend, and don't have time to give anything - let alone our purpose - a moment's thought. Or, you may still have faith in the dream that we each have a purpose, and you may have been searching and searching, but haven't figured out exactly what it is yet.

I have no doubt that your calling has been trying to connect with you, but you've made yourself so busy or so smothered with other things that you haven't been able to sense it. To help things along, find some quiet time alone each day – perhaps take the time to set up a regular meditation practice. During that time notice what draws you, what is pulling you toward it. It may help to repeat the question, "What is my purpose?" or "How can I serve?" It may take some time, but when the time is right you'll hear the call.

During your daily life notice what is grabbing your attention. Do you have a desire to learn to dance hip hop? Perhaps you tell yourself that it's too late to start now, or that you'll never be any good. Ignore those critical voices in your head and give it a go. Get some lessons. If you're struggling to discover your purpose, and we each have our own unique way to serve in the world, then try this little exercise.

Workbook Exercise: Purpose

Go to your workbook, but before you start, clear your mind. Get rid of any preconceptions you have about yourself and how the world should be. You will really need to take some quiet time here. Is your head clear? Are you ready to see yourself with new eyes? If you are, you are ready to go.

Answer this question: What is my true purpose?

Write any answer that pops into your head.

Repeat this step until you come to an answer that really resonates with you, you'll feel an emotional surge with it.

Just keep going until you get to something that feels right. For some of us it will take five minutes, for others half an hour or more. You may need to spend some time on it one day, take a break, and come back to it the next day. Persist until you get an answer with energy.

By the end of this section, I hope you are happy that you're in the best environment you can be – both at work and at home. Maybe you are opening up your world by exploring and being creative. And, I hope you haven't left out play – enjoy life, have some fun. The ultimate win will be if you have discovered your purpose or your meaning for being on this little world. This is a very difficult one to achieve, so don't feel too bad if you are still searching. Personally, I had to quit my career, and then travel and explore for almost a year before I finally found mine. It wasn't easy, and yet, when I found it, my purpose seemed so obvious; all the little bits and pieces I'd been playing at over the years finally coalesced into something of meaning. It's happening for you too, but it may not be obvious just yet.

PART IV

ESSENTIALS

16

IMPORTANT EXTRAS

This section covers four elements that I consider *essential* to authentic living. These four elements are: being present or staying in the now (mindfulness), gratitude, giving, and simplicity – our ability to un-complicate our lives. I highly recommend trying to integrate these elements into your everyday life.

17

BEING PRESENT

"To get the most success out of life have no agenda other than to give whatever you can in the present moment. A smile, a laugh, a quarter, a helping hand, an introduction or just your listening ear is more powerful than you can imagine. Beneath every gift is the knowing that the Universe is abundant and that you lose nothing by giving away what you have. Others will feel comfortable in your presence and all good things will find you – without seeking them."

~ Jackson Kiddard

I don't know about you, but I love this quote, I can read it over and over again without getting bored. Did you read and absorb it? Or did you just skim over it? Are you whizzing through this book as fast as you can? And is this how you live your life - racing through it to get as many things done as quickly as possible? Whether you read the quote above, or not, take a long slow breath, go back, and read it again, very slowly and with consideration. Don't worry, I'll wait.

Welcome back. Now, wasn't that a nice experience. Imagine if your whole life became full of such enriching experiences. Wouldn't it be truly wonderful? Everything would have more depth, more meaning, and would be so much more pleasurable. Being present is about mindfulness. It's about being aware of every moment. It's the key to living a full and satisfying life. When we are mindful we notice the little things. For example, imagine you are in a restaurant eating soup. Being mindful means noticing the taste of the soup you're consuming, the soup's temperature, the feeling of the liquid as it moves down into your stomach, the feeling of the nutrition you gain as it absorbs into your system. At the same time you notice the chair you are sitting on, is it hard or soft, is it stable or wobbly? What noises can you hear in the environment around you? What noises are close? What noises are coming from further away? When we are very mindful we notice all that is going on around us – the colours, the lights, the people near us. There is so much happening in our environment that we can too easily miss if we're not aware, or if we are caught up in our thinking, wandering mind.

I've mentioned this before and I'll mention it again, I've found there is an interesting paradox that occurs in relation to time as you become more mindful. I find that the more mindful I am, and the more I slow things down, the longer and more full my days seem to become. It's as though being aware, fully aware, of what is going on around me has effectively slowed time down. It's a wonderful experience. Life is no longer a race; it's slow, steady, vibrant, and full. And, surprisingly, I get even more done than I used to. Interesting isn't it, and worth a try?

18

GRATITUDE

"Acknowledging the good that you already have in your life is the foundation for all abundance."

~ *Eckhart Tolle*

Gratitude is an amazing attitude, when you focus on how much you have to be grateful for, your mood shifts positively, and you feel energised. Make it a daily routine and feel the mental health benefits it provides.

Research has found that gratitude, like other positive emotions, broadens the scope of thinking and enables increased flexibility and creativity, it also assists in coping with stress and adversity (Folkman and Moskowitz, 2000). One way to build our gratitude muscle is to start a gratitude journal. Below is a quote is from the master of positivity – Martin Seligman.

"Every night for the next week, set aside ten minutes before you go to sleep. Write down three things that went well today and why they went well. You may use a journal or your computer to write about the events, but it is important that you have a physical record of what you wrote. The three things need not be earthshaking in importance ("My husband picked up my favourite ice cream for dessert on the way home from work today"), but they can be important ("My sister just gave birth to a healthy baby boy").

Next to each positive event, answer the question "Why did this happen?" For example, if you wrote that your husband picked up ice cream, write "because my husband is really thoughtful sometimes" or "because I remembered to call him from work and remind him to stop by the grocery store." Or if you wrote, "My sister just gave birth to a healthy baby boy," you might pick as the cause ... "She did everything right during her pregnancy" (Seligman, 2011).

At the end of the week, see how you feel. If you find it's making a difference to your mood – then please keep doing it.

Workbook Exercise: Gratitude

What are you grateful for? List down what you are grateful for today. As suggested, try setting up a gratitude journal and write down three things that you are grateful for each day and why.

19

GIVING

"Happiness doesn't result from what we get, but from what we give."

~ Ben Carson

Giving is a joy, the more we give the happier we become. Giving shows we care, and caring about others is what makes life a pleasure. Giving is not only about money – we can also give our time, our ideas, and our energy. Sometimes reframing giving as little acts of kindness can help you to consider giving in a more positive light and can make the action of giving seem more achievable.

Workbook Exercise: Giving

Make a commitment to do one act of kindness each day for a week. This may feel like hard work to start with, but I won't be at all surprised if you end up enjoying this exercise so much that you'll continue with it after the week is complete.

List out the days of the week, and note down each act of giving, and at the end of the week review your actions to see how they made you feel.

- Day one:
- Day two:
- Day three:
- Day four:
- Day five:
- Day six:
- Day seven:

Some Giving Ideas:

- Pay for the person behind you on the toll-way.
- Let someone in front of you in the queue at your local shop.
- Visit someone who you know is lonely.
- Give someone an unexpected gift.
- Phone a friend who you haven't spoken to in a while.
- Compliment a stranger sincerely.
- Leave a book you have already finished somewhere for someone else to read.
- Take cakes, chocolates, or flowers to neighbours or a local senior citizen.
- Donate money to charity.
- Copy a favourite recipe and give it to a friend.

- Offer to babysit.
- Donate clothes to goodwill.
- Bake cookies for the office.
- Write anonymous happy post-it notes for people to find.

20

SIMPLICITY

"Life is really simple, but we insist on making it complicated."

~ Confucius

To me simplicity is the absence of complication. You may be wondering if it's really possible to have an absence of complication in a world that seems to have got ridiculously overcomplicated. I know it seems challenging, but it really is possible.

We humans seem to have a natural tendency to make things very complicated. To add to our natural tendency, we have got ourselves into the unfortunate situation where busyness has become a badge of honour. I swear if I hear one more person complain about how busy they are, especially when they seem to be spending half their life on Facebook, I will scream. We decide to be busy – we do not have to be busy. We are the ones adding the busyness and drama to our lives. You may not want to hear it, but really, we are!

It is now the cultural norm, not just to *have* it all, but to *fit it all in*. Schulte (2014) mentions a researcher calling this obsession an exhausting 'every-day-athon', where we pack in a multitude of activities, socialising, and work obligations. Physicians are starting to call the modern drive toward fast-paced busyness a pathology, sometimes calling it 'time-sickness.' Psychologists write of treating burned-out clients who can't shake the notion that the busier they are, the more they are thought of as competent, smart, successful, admired, and even envied (Schulte, 2014).

Now, I know you are way too clever to get caught up in the busyness epidemic in such a bad way. However, it is easy to get caught up with a bit of day-to-day busy-ness, and sometimes we need to put a little bit of effort into reducing the busy-ness and making life simpler. Below are a few easy tricks to get you on the road to simpler living.

1. **Spend less.** Do you really need that new dress, that new pair of shoes, that new gadget? What if you saved that money? How much freedom could it give you in the long run? The next time you're considering purchasing an item, think about whether the old version of it is really fully used up. Are those old sneakers really not doing the job any more? Or, are you just getting sucked in to buying a new pair because they're new, they've been well marketed, and well, they just look fancier?

2. **Own less.** The more you own, the more it costs you. Own a fancy pair of shoes? What happens when the sole wears out and you need a new one? It will cost you to get it re-heeled. And what about TVs? How many TVs do you have in your household? Do you have a TV in every room? As well as encouraging antisocial behaviour (everyone in his or her own room watching the television), it is completely unnecessary, and, yes I'm

going to say it, excessive consumerism. Do I need to mention that it can be very expensive to get electrical items fixed these days. We're living in a disposable society – we buy things, they break, we throw them away, and then we buy more new things. It's not good for the environment, nor for our wallets. Too many of us are caught up in a cycle of purchasing new stuff and constant upgrading. De-cluttering can also help with simplification and the reduction of replacement or repair costs. Is it time for a spring-clean? What do you have in your house that you haven't used for a few months or even years. When I de-cluttered my apartment recently, because I was moving homes, I found some brand new items that I'd purchased two years ago and had never used. Yes, I'm guilty too! I ended up selling them, and wondered why I'd kept them for so long in the first place.

3. **Live in a small space.** When I lived in New Zealand I lived in a big old house all by myself. From New Zealand I moved to Asia, where I lived in a small apartment. You'd think the reduction in space might have been depressing, but I must admit that I loved the change. I didn't need so much space, I didn't need so much stuff, and it certainly helped to limit my spending. Because it was a serviced apartment it was fully furnished, so I didn't have any repair costs for any household goods, ever. Perfect! Another benefit of this rapidly changing world is that now there are some great designs for small houses. People from all walks of life are finding ways to live in smaller spaces that are cheaper to build. Why don't you join this exciting new trend and downsize your living space?

4. **The power of a word.** Words are a critical part of how we express ourselves. Sometimes we forget that the

words we use has a big impact on others. It is very rare that we speak with full awareness, and with the objective of keeping things simple. Do we really think about what are we trying to say? Are we using the right words? Are we saying something useful or just talking for the sake of talking? One thing I learnt at a recent meditation retreat is the power of trying to focus thoughts down to only a few words. This process increases your awareness of what you're saying and ensures you communicate more succinctly. The next time you have something to say, before you speak, ask yourself if your thought can be expressed in a few key words. Give it a try – it's certainly challenging, but also very powerful.

5. **Unsubscribe.** We all get inundated with way too much information these days. One helpful way to reduce the influx of unnecessary information is to unsubscribe from anything that no longer serves us. Are there postal deliveries that you can change to online deliveries? When you get phone calls from unsolicited callers, ask to be removed from their database. Clean up your email subscriptions. If you get something you love, then register for a weekly update rather than daily. We sign up to so many seemingly useful emails, but ask yourself, how many of these emails do you actually read, and how many do you realistically need? As an old boss of mine used to say, a clear desk is a sign of a clear mind – I guess the same is true of your inbox.

After completing this section have you found that you are living increasingly in the present? Take the time to investigate meditation and mindfulness practices to help in this area. Are you feeling grateful more regularly? Have you established your own gratitude journaling practice? I hope you enjoyed the giving exercise, it can be a lot of fun, both for you and those you interact with, make it game, and keep playing it for as long as you can. And finally, I hope you've been able to take the time to simplify your life as much as possible. Getting rid of the clutter in our lives helps to reduce the clutter in our minds.

PART V

A LITTLE MORE INSPIRATION

21

NEXT STEPS

"Faith is taking the first step even when you don't see the whole staircase."

~ *Martin Luther King, Jr.*

Well done for completing this journey, I hope you've enjoyed it. You may well be asking yourself, what now? Relax and enjoy what you've learnt. Keep your workbook close at hand, review it regularly, and gradually implement the changes you've decided to make. Don't try to do everything all at once, just pick one thing at a time to try, change, or implement.

Keep in mind that life is a big adventure, and you're the hero of your own personal quest. You only need to ensure you're on the right path and the rest will follow easily and smoothly.

I've included some additional resources in the following section to keep you inspired and on track. Please contact me with your thoughts, feedback, and input on the process and your own personal journey at sarah@sarahoflaherty.com. The best thing about writing is interacting with my readers.

I wish you all the best and thank you for taking part in this magical adventure.

22

INSPIRATION

"Goals. There's no telling what you can do when you get inspired by them. There's no telling what you can do when you believe in them. There's no telling what will happen when you act upon them."

~ Jim Rohn

"The most absurd and reckless aspirations have sometimes led to extraordinary success."

~ Vauvenargues

"Through generosity, we cultivate a generous spirit. Generosity of spirit will usually lead to generosity of action, but being a generous

person is more important than any particular act of giving. After all, it is possible to give without it's being a generous act."

~ Gil Fronsdal, The Joy of Giving

'The excessive emphasis on the fast-paced instant way of life is undoubtedly the most dangerous enemy of joy. As much as possible, as fast as possible, is its motto. It leads to more and more fun, and less and less joy."

~ Hermann Hesse

"Use what talents you possess, for the woods would be very quiet if no birds sang there except those that sang best."

~ Henry Van Dyke

"Remember, happiness doesn't depend on who you are or what you have; it depends solely on what you think."

~ Dale Carnegie

"Life is a great big canvas, and you should throw all the paint on it you can."

~ Danny Kaye

"Though no one can go back and make a brand new start, anyone can start now and make a brand new ending."

~ Carl Bard

"Enjoy the little things, for one day you may look back and realise they were the big things."

~ Robert Brault

"Winners are losers who got up and gave it one more try."

~ Dennis Deyoung

"Life is like riding a bicycle. To keep your balance you must keep moving."

~ Albert Einstein

"The highest reward for a person's toil is not what they get for it, but what they become by it."

~ *John Ruskin*

"The best preparation for tomorrow is to do today's work superbly well."

~ *Sir William Osler*

"You can complain because roses have thorns, or you can rejoice because thorns have roses."

~ *Ziggy*

"Success is the ability to go from failure to failure without losing your enthusiasm."

~ *Sir Winston Churchill*

"Our life is what our thoughts make of it."

~ *Marcus Aurelius*

Some books are life changing; they somehow shift you up a level. We all have different tastes and needs, however, I wanted to share with you some of the books that have made a difference to my life.

Choose Yourself. By James Altucher

Reason for Hope: A Spiritual Journey. By Jane Goodall

The Element: How Finding Your Passion Changes Everything. By Ken Robinson

Love Yourself Like Your Life Depends On It. By Kamal Ravikant

The Four Agreements: A Practical Guide to Personal Freedom. By Miguel Ruiz

Loving What Is: Four Questions That Can Change Your Life. By Byron Katie

Too Nice For Your Own Good: How To Stop Making 9 Self-Sabotaging Mistakes. By Duke Robinson

7 Habits of Highly Effective People: Powerful Lessons In Personal Change. By Stephen R. Covey

Flow, The Psychology of Optimal Experience. By Mihaly Csikszentmihaly

Quiet: The Power of Introverts in a World That Can't Stop Talking. By Susan Cain

The Man Who Planted Trees. By Jean Giono

The Alchemist. By Paulo Coehlo

Mans Search For Meaning. By Victor E. Frankl

The Celestine Prophesy. By James Redfield

Outliers: The Story of Success. By Malcolm Gladwell

Tipping Point: How Little Things Can Make a Big Difference. By Malcolm Gladwell

A Joseph Campbell Companion: Reflections on the Art of Living. By Joseph Campbell

Myths to Live By. By Joseph Campbell

Siddhartha. By Hermann Hesse

The Seasons of the Soul. By Hermann Hesse

The Power of Now. By Eckhart Tolle

The Seat of the Soul. By Gary Zukav

The Go-Giver: A Little Story About a Powerful Business Idea. By Bob Burg

The End of Your World. By Adyashanti

Clean Gut: The Breakthrough Plan. By Alejandro Junger

The Wise Heart: A Guide to the Universal Teachings of Buddhist Psychology. By Jack Kornfield

Game of Life and How to Play It. By Florence Scovel Shinn

How to Make a Journal of Your Life. By Dan Price

These days there are also some great websites we can use to inspire us. Here are a couple that I recommend you take the time to check out:

www. zenpencils.com

"Gavin Aung Than is a freelance cartoonist based in Melbourne, Australia. After working in the corporate graphic design industry for eight years he quit his unfulfilling job at the end of 2011 to focus on his true passion, drawing cartoons. Gavin launched *Zen Pencils* at the start of 2012, a cartoon blog which adapts inspirational quotes into comic stories, and he hasn't looked back since."

www.thepowerofless.com

"With the countless distractions that come from every corner of modern life, it's amazing that we're ever able to accomplish anything. The Power of Less demonstrates how to streamline your life by identifying the essential and eliminating the unnecessary - freeing you from everyday clutter and allowing you to focus on accomplishing the goals that can change your life for the better."

12 STEPS TO SELF CARE

1. If it feels wrong, don't do it
2. Say exactly what you mean
3. Don't be a people pleaser
4. Trust your instincts
5. Never speak badly about yourself
6. Never give up on your dreams
7. Don't be afraid to say 'No'
8. Don't be afraid to say 'Yes'
9. Be kind to yourself
10. Let go of what you can't control
11. Stay away from drama and negativity
12. LOVE

VIP CLUB

Building a relationship with my readers is something I love about writing. I occasionally send out newsletters with information on upcoming books, recommended books to read, life improvement tools, and great daily rituals.

If you join my VIP Club I'll send you the following free:

1. Values Online Lesson
2. The Simplify Your Life Workbook
3. 12 Steps to Self-Care Poster

Click to join my VIP Club
http://bit.ly/sylsarah

PLEASE LEAVE A REVIEW

Enjoy this book? You can make a big difference

Reviews are the most powerful tools I have when it comes to getting attention for my books. Much as I'd like to, I don't have the financial muscle of a New York publisher. I can't take out full page ads in the newspaper or put up billboard posters

(Not yet, anyway).

But I do have something much more powerful and effective than that, and it's something those publishers would kill to get their hands on.

A committed and loyal bunch of readers.

Honest reviews of my books help bring them to the attention of other readers.

If you've enjoyed this book I would be very grateful if you could spend just five minutes leaving a review (it can be as short as you like). You can find your preferred store by simply clicking below.

Simplify Your Life

Thank you very much.

ABOUT THE AUTHOR

Sarah has extensive experience in leadership, people management, mediation, and working with change. She is also the author of Ready For A Career Change. Sarah's online home is www.sarahoflaherty.com. You can connect with Sarah on Twitter at @sarahof, and on Facebook at www.facebook.com/sarahoflahertymind and you can send her an email at sarah@sarahoflaherty.com if you ever feel so inclined.

·

MORE BOOKS FROM SARAH

Ready For A Career Change

Feeling trapped in a job you don't like? Discover how to transition into a new career with learnings from people who've done it.

Working long hours, with no satisfaction? Want to start your own business, but not sure you can? Changing careers or setting up your own business isn't easy. Let experienced career coach Sarah O'Flaherty show you how others have made the transition.

Sarah O'Flaherty has a successful business assisting people to improve their job/life satisfaction and to work through career transition. After a successful twenty-year career in advertising, Sarah is now training to become a Clinical Psychologist. Using her own experience and interviews with others who have made major changes or established their own businesses, Sarah has created 9 landmark questions to get you through a career change in one piece. By answering these questions, you'll ensure a transition with minimal stress, while maintaining your relationships, your home, and your sanity.

Inside *Ready for a Career Change?* you'll discover:

• How to break down the barriers we face when changing jobs so you can make the best decision for you.

• How others have changed careers and their key learnings so you can save time and benefit from their experience.

• The important questions to consider in a career change so you don't waste your time and energy on something that's not right for you.

• The benefits of a career change, such as increased energy and job satisfaction.

• And much, much more!

Ready for a Career Change? Is packed with straightforward, honest, and practical advice that can be your wake-up call to the life that awaits you in a new career. If you like easy reads that tell it to you straight, then you'll love having Sarah on your team.

Ready for a Career Change?

∾

Fresh Start: A Guide To Eliminating Unhealthy Stress

Feeling overwhelmed? Do you have trouble sleeping? Are you feeling increasingly depressed? Could you be suffering from burnout? We all experience stress, but sometimes stress can leave us physically and emotionally drained. It can be difficult to regain a sense of balance in our lives.

Inside *Fresh Start – A Guide to Eliminating Unhealthy Stress* you'll discover:

• What stress is, so that you can understand whether you're affected.

- The difference between stress and burnout, so that you know which of these you're dealing with.

- The many sources of stress, the key triggers, and how to halt stress in its tracks.

- Different coping strategies, so that you can see how your current coping strategies might be modified for better results

- In the moment stress reduction strategies, so that you can lower your stress levels today.

- And much, much more!

There are answers. Discover how to manage unhealthy stress and start feeling more calm and peaceful. Let Sarah O'Flaherty guide you to a healthier, happier life.

Sarah O'Flaherty assists people in improving their job/life satisfaction, and working through career transitions. Currently training as a clinical psychologist, Sarah leverages the latest research and techniques for managing unhealthy stress to help her clients emerge from the chaos of stress and find balance and greater peace in their lives. In *Fresh Start*, Sarah teaches you about stress in any easy to understand format, with the hope of releasing you from damaging stress once and for all. *Fresh Start* will help you to transition away from stress, while maintaining your relationships, your job, your home, and your sanity.

Fresh Start is packed with straightforward, honest, and practical advice that can be your wake-up call to a new start in life. If you like easy reads that tell it to you straight, then you'll love having Sarah on your team.

Buy *A Fresh Start* to help you return to calm and balanced living!

Purchase:

Amazon US

Amazon UK

Amazon AU

For more information:
www.sarahoflaherty.com

Many thanks to all those that assisted me in this process, they include:

Mark Dawson and team, Lynn and Dennis Ryan, Stuart Bache

Start by doing what's necessary; then do what's possible; suddenly you are doing the impossible.

—Francis of Assisi

APPENDIX: VALUES LIST

Abundance

Acceptance

Accessibility

Accomplishment

Accuracy

Achievement

Acknowledgement

Adaptability

Adoration

Adroitness

Adventure

Affection

Affluence

Aggressiveness

Agility

Alertness

Altruism

Ambition

Amusement

Anticipation

Appreciation

Approachability

Articulacy

Assertiveness

Assurance

Attentiveness

Attractiveness

Audacity

Availability

Awareness

Awe

Balance

Beauty

Being the best

Belonging

Benevolence

Bliss

Boldness

Bravery

Brilliance

Buoyancy

Calmness

Camaraderie

Candor

Capability

Care

Carefulness

Celebrity

Certainty

Challenge

Charity

Charm

Chastity

Cheerfulness

Clarity

Cleanliness

Cleverness

Closeness

Comfort

Commitment

Compassion

Completion

Composure

Concentration

Confidence

Conformity

Congruency

Connection

Consciousness

Consistency

Contentment

Continuity

Contribution

Control

Conviction

Conviviality

Coolness

Cooperation

Cordiality

Correctness

Courage

Courtesy

Craftiness

Creativity

Credibility

Cunning

Curiousity

Daring

Decisiveness

Decorum

Deference

Delight

Depth

Dependability

Determination

Devotion

Devoutness

Dexterity

Desire

Dignity

Diligence

Direction

Directness

Discipline

Discovery

Discretion

Diversity

Dominance

Dreaming

Drive

Duty

Dynamism

Eagerness

Economy

Ecstasy

Education

Effectiveness

Efficiency

Elation

Elegance

Empathy

Encouragement

Endurance

Energy

Enjoyment

Entertainment

Enthusiasm

Excellence

Excitement

Exhiliration

Expectancy

Expediency

Experience

Expertise

Exploration

Expressiveness

Extravagance

Extroversion

Exuberance

Fairness

Faith

Fame

Family

Fascination

Fashion

Fearlessness

Ferocity

Fidelity

Fierceness   .

Firmness

Fitness

Flexibility

Flow

Fluency

Focus

Fortitude

Frankness

Freedom

Friendliness

Frugality

Fun

Gallantry

Generosity

Gentility

Giving

Grace

Gratitude

Gregariousness

Growth

Guidance

Happiness

Harmony

Health

Heart

Helpfulness

Heroism

Holiness

Honesty

Honor

Hopefulness

Hospitality

Humility

Hunour

Hygiene

Imagination

Impact

Impartiality

Independence

Industry

Ingenuity

Inquisitiveness

Insightful

Inspiration

Integrity

Intelligence

Intensity

Intimacy

Intrepidness

Introversion

Intuition

Intuitiveness

Investing

Inventiveness

Joy

Judiciousness

Justice

Keenness

Kindness

Knowledge

Leadership

Learning

Liberation

Liberty

Liveliness

Logic

Longevity

Love

Loyalty

Majesty

Mastery

Maturity

Meekness

Mellowness

Meticulousness

Mindfulness

Modesty

Motivation

Mysteriousness

Neatness

Nerve

Obedience

Openminded

Openness

Optimism

Order

Organisation

Originality

Outlandishness

Outrageousness

Passion

Peace

Perceptiveness

Perfection

Perkiness

Perseverance

Persistence

Persuasiveness

Philanthropy

Piety

Playfulness

Pleasantness

Pleasure

Poise

Polish

Popularity

Potency

Power

Practicality

Pragmatism

Precision

Preparedness

Presence

Privacy

Proactivity

Professionalism

Prosperity

Prudence

Punctuality

Purity

Realism

Reason

Reasonableness

Recognition

Recreation

Refinement

Reflection

Relaxation

Reliability

Religiousness

Resilience

Resolution

Resolve

Resourcefulness

Respect

Rest

Restraint

Reverence

Richness

Rigor

Sacredness

Sacrifice

Sagacity

Saintliness

Sanguinity

Satisfaction

Security

Self-control

Selflessness

Self-reliance

Sensitivity

Sensuality

Serenity

Service

Sexuality

Sharing

Shrewdness

Significance

Silence

Stillness

Simplicity

Sincerity

Skillfulness

Solidarity

Solitude

Soundness

Speed

Spirit

Spirituality

Spontaneity

Spunk

Stability

Stealth

Stillness

Strength

Structure

Success

Support

Supremacy

Surprise

Sympathy

Synergy

Teamwork

Temperance

Thankfulness

Thoroughness

Thoughtfulness

Thrift

Tidiness

Timeliness

Traditionalism

Tranquility

Transcendence

Trust

Trustworthiness

Truth

Understanding

Unflappability

Uniqueness

Unity

Usefulness

Utility

Valor

Variety

Victory

Vigor

Virtue

Vision

Vitality

Vivacity

Warmth

Watchfulness

Wealth

Willfulness

Willingness

Winning

Wisdom

Wittiness

Wonder

Youthfulness

Zeal

REFERENCES

Andrews P, Benbrook C, Davies N, et al. (2008) New Evidence Confirms the Nutritional Superiority of Plant-Based Organic Foods. *State of Science Review.* The Organic Centre: University of Arizona.

Berman MG, Jonides J and Kaplan S. (2008) The Cognitive Benefits of Interacting With Nature. *Psychological Science* 19: 1207-1212.

Bowler DE, Buyung-Ali LM, Knight TM, et al. (2010) A systematic review of evidence for the added benefits to health of exposure to natural environments. *BMC Public Health* 10: 456-456.

Csikszentmihalyi M. (1990) *Flow,* New York: Harper & Row.

de Botton A. (2014) The News: A User's Manual. In: de Botton A (ed) *Ideas at the House.* Sydney Opera House.

Folkman S and Moskowitz JT. (2000) Positive affect and the other side of coping. *American Psychologist* 55: 647-654.

Rieber LP. (1996) Seriously Considering Play: Designing Interactive Learning Environments Based on the Blending of

Microworlds, Simulations, and Games. *Educational Technology Research and Development* 44: 43-58.

Schulte B. (2014) *Overwhelmed,* London: Bloomsbury Publishing.

Seligman M. (2011) *Flourish,* New York: Free Press.